Mind Games For Consenting Adults

The Definitive Guide To Bedroom Hypnosis

Dr. Randall L. Maynard
Certified Clinical Hypnotherapist

Attitude 1

7092 Agatha Drive

Stokesdale, North Carolina

27357

(336) 644-0889
(336) 509-1125

Nordique_1@msn.com

www.attitude1.net

Dedicated to enhancing and sustaining relationships.

ISBN13: 978-0-6151-4079-7

Index

Index (Continued)

Preface

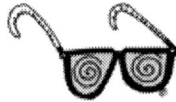

Relax. Relax. Relax. Relax. Relax.

Congratulations! Now you know the secret of Hypnosis!

"Hypno" is derived from the Greek meaning sleep, or relax.

Hypnosis is a Heightened State of Relaxation.

You do not have to look deep into my eyes as I swing a golden watch while inducing or seducing you with some surrealistic Transylvanian voice.

All you need is a quiet environment and a place to make yourself comfortable.

So, what's the trick?

It is believed that we only use 8 to 12 percent of our minds. The remaining 88 to 92 percent is regarded as inaccessible worthless gray matter.

This could not be farther from the truth.

Basically, we have several cerebral layers:

The conscious (that 8-12% previously noted), subconscious (just below the surface, lurking in your dreams, etc.), and the unconscious (the knower). We, as humans, have a tendency to exist primarily in the conscious level due to our lives, jobs, relationships, etc.

Consciously, we rarely have enough capacity to control ourselves as we know we should. We get tense, we smoke, become excessively inhibited, lose our zest for life, etc.

If we could improve our skills and abilities or modify our behavior quickly and safely, then why shouldn't we?

Hypnosis is safe and effective. The inductions and suggestions provided in this book are totally safe. You may feel confident trusting your partner to share this experience with you. You can NOT be hypnotized to do anything, which would not be morally or ethically acceptable to you. The worst that you may expect is to have a very pleasant period of rest and relaxation.

You have already been hypnotized dozens, hundreds, maybe even thousands of times. Have you ever been driving down the interstate only to find you have been in a daze for the last 30 miles? How about those times you zoned out while staring at the television? Each of these times constituted entry into the hypnotic state or a heightened state of relaxation.

The entire process revolves around relaxation and subconscious suggestion. Despite the simplicity of its' nature, there is a lot more to it than is exhibited in stage shows and smoking clinics.

An entire universe of mental, physical, and spiritual growth can be found in its usage.

The concept I have chosen for this book is to show you than in your own family room or bedroom, you can change your life.

This "toy" can help your marriage, improve your golf game, get better grades for your children, help you loose weight, quit smoking, have better sex...virtually ANYTHING you can imagine!

The best part is YOU CAN DO IT YOURSELF!

...or, you may continue paying people like myself $75 to $200 per hour to do it for you!

My favorite part about Hypnosis is that I don't have to spend two hours a day, every day, practicing relaxation techniques or doing body positioning in order to keep my head on straight.

It is quick, easy, painless, safe, and requires only about 15 to 30 minutes per session, AND, it does not have to be done every day.

I am elated with what Hypnosis has done for my life, and I hope it will have the same positive impact on yours.

Introduction

This book/program was conceived for couples. A minimum of two people is required.

Ideally, your partner is or will become you best friend, mentor, playmate, support group, teammate, lover, and soul mate long before you complete this program.

Try this IF…

You have forgotten how to talk to each other…
If you are too busy to play…
If you want some safe fun that can be achieved in a reasonable time frame…
If you want to add another dimension to your relationship…
If you want to change your life for the better…
Or if you just want new subject matter for that digital camera you just acquired!

Your nights will never be the same!

This book consists of a collection of hypnotic inductions, suggestions, and experiences…all discovered in the comfort of my own bedroom and family room.

This all came about after seeing Mike Harvey's Hypnotist show at a local comedy club in Lake Charles, Louisiana way back in 1979. (He was incredible!)

I absolutely had to learn more about the reality of Hypnosis!

I tried calling numerous local practitioners only to find that they wanted $500 or more to teach this skill to me.

A quick trip to the library and local bookstores left me with an abundance of literature, and believe it or not, within a couple of hours, I was practicing my first session with my partner.

When we discovered that the first suggestion I tried on her worked, there was no stopping the quest.

I would never have believed at that time that enough material would arise from this curiosity to fill an entire book and have a blast doing it.

Throughout this book, I have tried to guide and prepare you as well as possible without becoming overly clinical. I also have tried to share any apprehensions I have discovered which accompany the powers of Hypnosis.

You will NOT believe how much fun this can be!

A Note of Caution

If you have Physical Symptoms or Emotional issues which are either prolonged or severe, please consult a Physician or Therapist and get the okay to go ahead prior to attempting to "heal" your self with this book.

The Author disclaims any liabilities that may arise from the use or misuse of this book and its contents.

How It Works

The elements of Hypnosis are each very logical. One is GUIDED into relaxing by use of breathing techniques, visualization, and the influence of soft music and a calm voice (progressive relaxation)
.

Once relaxation has been maximized, suggestions are made in a positive manner that will in some way improve or enhance the life and/or mindset of the "client". Once the suggestion(s) has been made, the client is brought gently back into a state of conscious awareness, feeling refreshed and relaxed.

The following section is a complete session as it would be done in the office of a Certified Hypnotherapist. Try reading/practicing it in a patient and gentle manner. It is specifically designed to lower ones anxiety level. If you read it, word for word, to your partner in the presence of a quiet atmosphere, possibly adding soft music or ocean sounds and candlelight, you will find it is flawlessly effective. So, let's get started!

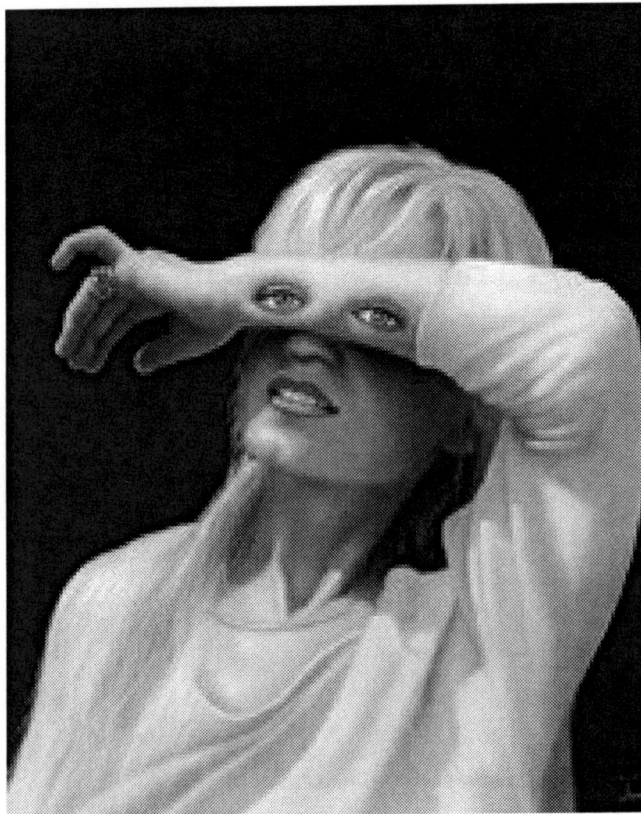

A Complete Session:

Anxiety Management
Induction and Script

Take a few minutes to insure privacy and quiet for the next hour.
Turn down or off the lights.
Cut off your telephones.
Put on a relaxing CD, ocean sounds, etc., at low volume.
Make sure you will be completely undisturbed.

Choose a favorite recliner; adjust your volume, Light incense or a candle.

Make sure you can be totally comfortable.

Now, settle into your chair, relax, and accept that for the next hour or so you have nowhere to go and nothing to do.

Here is where you began the induction and script...you may read it word for word:

For the next hour you will be guided by my voice.
Concentrating only on my voice
Let no outside sounds disturb you
Any sounds you hear will only help you to relax more deeply

Let the music move into the very soul of your existence
Let it take you away

Now, Just relax.
Think about what the letters R E L A X mean to you.
Let go.
Relax.

Now take in a deep breath through your nose.
Hold it in while you mentally count to 5.
During this count, gather up all your tensions and frustrations and on the count of 5, strongly exhale them through your mouth.
And relax.
Just relax.

Lets repeat the breathing exercise.

Deep breath in through your nose.
Hold while you count to 5.
Gather up anything that should not be a part of you.
And blow it out through your mouth.

Relax.

Just relax.

Let your breathing become gentle and rhythmic.

Just relax.

Let your body settle gently into your chair, uncross your legs, let the chair support every inch of your physical body.

Relax.

Feel your self sink into the cushions and relax.

Now bring the center of your concentration to your left foot and relax your left foot.
Completely relax your left foot.
Every muscle, tendon, ligament, nerve ending and every molecule.
Completely relax your left foot.

Just relax your left foot.

Now feel the relaxation move up through your ankle, your calf, your knee, your thigh, and into your hip…and relax.

Just relax.

Next, concentrate on you Right foot.
Completely relax your right foot.
Every muscle, tendon, ligament, nerve ending and every molecule.
Completely relax your right foot.

Just relax.

Notice that the entire lower half of your body is now very relaxed and comfortable.
Let it sink into the cushions as you relax.

Now, focus on your lower back.
Your lower back has a tendency to harbor tensions and anxieties.
Let these tensions move out and away from your lower back as you relax.
Relax your lower back.
Deeply.
Completely.
Relax your lower back.

Now, let the relaxation move up your spine.
And as it goes up your vertebrae, it is as if a pair of magical massage hands are kneading each muscle in your back, massaging you, helping you to relax.

And finally the relaxation reaches the back of your neck.
Relax your neck.
Allow the tensions that have found refuge there to move away
And completely relax the back of your neck.
Just relax.

And the relaxation moves up the back of your head, across your scalp, and down over your forehead.
Smoothing out the little worry lines.
Allowing you to relax even deeper.
Relax the little muscles around your eyes.
Just relax.
Part your teeth slightly.
Relax your jaw.
Relax.
Let go.

And the relaxation moves down over your chest, stomach, and abdomen.
Although you are completely relaxed, your organs will continue to function properly, helping you to relax more and more deeply.

Just relax.

Now concentrate on your left shoulder.
Relax your left shoulder.
Every tendon, ligament, nerve ending, and molecule.
Totally relax your left shoulder.
Relax.
Let the relaxation flow down through your upper arm, your elbow, your forearm, your wrist, into your hand, your fingers, and your thumb.
Just relax.
Relax.

Next, concentrate on your right shoulder.

Relax your right shoulder.
Every tendon, ligament, nerve ending, and molecule.
Completely relax your right shoulder.
Relax.
Let the relaxation flow down through your upper arm, your elbow, your forearm, your wrist, into your hand, your fingers, and your thumb.
Just relax.

Let go.

Imagine a wave of relaxation flowing through you from the top of your head to the bottom of your feet.

Just let go.
Just relax.

Now I want you to use the power of your imagination to picture a beautiful downward spiraling staircase in front of you.
Covered is soft thick luxurious carpet.
Winding down with 10 steps.
In a moment, we are going to descend this staircase together.
As we do, I will count backward from 10 to 1 with each descending number taking you deeper down into relaxation.

Let us take our first step down
10
Relax
You can physically feel yourself going down
9
Stepping down, relaxing deeper down
8
Down
Gently down, more deeply relaxed.
7
Just let go and relax as you continue going deeper into relaxation
6
Down, safely, comfortably down
5
Relax
Just relax
4
Deeper relaxed than you have ever been
Going down now to
3
Relax
2

Just completely let yourself relax
1
Where you find yourself more relaxed than you have ever been.

And now you find there is a door in front of you.
Opening the door, you see a beautiful beach outside.
As you step through the door,
You find yourself on a private Caribbean island
On a beautiful day
With the warm sun caressing your skin
And you are so relaxed.
Feel the sand under your feet as you walk along the beach
So safe
So secure
No one to disturb you
On this beautiful day
Somewhere in the Caribbean.
You can feel the gentle breeze against your skin
And taste the salt in the air.
You hear the seagulls in the distance
And you relax
Relax
And as you wander down the beach you find a hammock
Put there just for you.
See yourself gently safely climbing into the hammock
So comfortable
So warm
So safe
So content
And you find yourself rocking gently
Back and forth
Back and forth
So very relaxed
No where to go
Nothing to do but relax
Rocking
Back and forth
Back and forth

There is a trash bag beside the hammock
Pick it up
Begin to reach inside yourself and pull out all things in you that should not be part of
your being
Pull out angers, frustrations, resentments, tensions, and anxieties
What ever is in you that should not be, pull it out and put it in the bag

I am going to be silent for a moment so you can fill your bag
Relax

Now, closing the bag, you can see it magically begin to rise up
The higher it rises, the smaller it appears to be
Until it disappears
Along will all of the garbage that used to be part of you

And you relax
Just relax

As you continue to rock back and forth, breathing gently, so relaxed and comfortable
I want you to see your inner spiritual self, rising safely and comfortably above your physical self
To a point about 100 feet in the air
As you reach this point, I want you to completely relax and let go

As you look down upon your physical self,
You can see the real you
You can also see the future you

There is a miraculous change about to take place in you
A tingling sensation warms your spirit as you anxiously await these changes

Relax

This pleasant relaxed experience you are having now will gradually come to be characteristic of you.
See yourself going about your daily life with confident composure and a feeling of inner calm.
Whenever something happens that causes you to feel tension, temporarily stop what you are doing, inhale deeply, and then slowly exhale.
As you exhale, you will experience an inner calm and feel a sense of confident composure as it flows through your body.

As you look down upon your physical self, you can see yourself transformed into a relaxed and confident individual.
You can feel closely the problems with the old self as they pass through you
These negatives rise up from your physical body
Pass through your spiritual self
And disappear into space and time

As these feelings pass through you
You rejoice internally

Relax

Just relax in your newfound happiness and sense of well-being

Relax

Now, I want you to slowly descend back into your physical body
Gently settling down and in
Like a hand slipping into a glove.

Relax

Breathing gently and rhythmically

Just relax

In a moment I am going to count from one to five with five being wide awake

When you awaken, you will feel clean, confident, relaxed and ready to take on the world

Relax

You are free from feelings of tension and anxiety.
You are powerful.
 You have made a decision to control your life and it begins NOW

1
2 beginning to wake up
3 waking up, opening your eyes
4 opening you eyes now
5 wide awake, refreshed, relaxed, and comfortable

Take your time coming back into this moment
Lie there and enjoy the music

You may get up whenever you feel like doing so

The session is now complete. The subject will not feel as though they have been hypnotized, of course. Just remember, it is a heightened state of relaxation. Do they feel relaxed?

Induction Techniques

This section exhibits Induction Techniques, a very critical component of Hypnosis. The four major elements of successful Hypnosis are as follows:

1. Instill confidence in your "subject"
2. Put them into a trance (induction)
3. Modify their behavior (suggestion)
4. Wake them up

And you thought this was complicated, didn't you?

First, in a calm soothing voice, slowly read verbatim the induction scripts of your choice to your subject.

Next, turn to the suggestion script of your choice, and read it to your subject in the same manner as the induction.

Each suggestion is ended with the upward count, which brings the person to the waking state. If you wish for the suggestion to be left with that person than you are now finished.

If you are "playing" and wish to remove the imposed trance/suggestion, simply have your subject relax again by counting backwards from ten to one, and tell them they are no longer in the state in which you left them. (Don't confuse them by suggesting they are now in Wyoming!)

It is best to review it and practice it first so that no stumbling will occur during the induction/suggestion process.

It is not necessary for a suggestion to be lengthy for it to be effective, so you will find several of the provided suggestions to be rather short. Remember to use only ONE suggestion per induction, lest you confuse your subject.

It is also a good idea to take this process seriously, even if you are playing, and above all else pay attention!

Hypnosis is safe, but be sure you consider the impact and consequences of the suggestion prior to administering it.

Bon voyage and Good Luck!

Quick Induction Technique

Make yourself comfortable.
Take a deep breath, and relax.
Just relax.
Take another deep breath, and as you exhale, let go of all your tensions and frustrations
And relax
Just relax

Relax your feet
Relax your lower legs
Relax your upper legs
Let go and allow your legs to completely relax

Relax your lower back
Relax your lower back
Feel the relaxation travel up your spine to your neck
Relax your neck and your back
Just relax
Completely relax

Listening only to my voice
Relax

Completely relax

Relax the muscles in your jaw
Relax the muscles in your face
Relax your eyes
Relax your scalp
Just relax
Completely relax

Let no outside sounds disturb you
Relax
Just relax

Imagine yourself on an elevator on the 10th floor
I am going to count backwards from 10 to 1
With each descending number taking you down another floor
And down another level of relaxation
Until you reach the first floor
Where you will find total relaxation

Feel yourself in the elevator now...10
You can feel it began to move gently downward....9
As you relax even deeper it reaches 8
Then 7, deeper down and more relaxed
Now 6, deeper into relaxation
More relaxed than ever before
5...going deeper and deeper down
4 ...even deeper than you have ever known
3...deeper down
2 ...just relax
1...completely relaxed
Totally relaxed and comfortable
Safely drifting and floating in a state of relaxation
Relaxed
Drifting
Floating
Just relax

(At this point you go to the suggestion of your choosing)

Sitting Induction

Sit back.
Uncross your legs.
Close your eyes.
Relax

Now, begin breathing deeply.
Take five deep breaths

With every breath you exhale, you will become more deeply relaxed.

After the fifth breath, concentrate on the weight of your shoes. Your shoes, being foreign to your normal body weight, will begin to feel heavy, and this heavy relaxation from your toes to your heels to your ankles will become very prominent.

You are now feeling this heavy relaxation moving upward into the calves of your legs...

Feeling the weight of your legs pushing down, heavier and heavier...

And feeling your legs relaxing deeply...

Deeply relaxing.

And this heavy relaxation moves into the knees, as you concentrate only on my voice.

Pay no attention to any outside sounds, hearing only my voice. These outside sounds are everyday sounds of life and cannot distract or disturb you. They will only tend to relax you and allow you to go even deeper into this deep, heavy relaxation.

Now feel the relaxation moving upward into your thighs and hips and through the midsection of your body…
Feel the stomach muscles relaxing…
Deeply relaxing…
And the entire chest area becomes saturated with relaxation.

Breathing becomes very deep

Gentle

Rhythmic

The drowsy, sleepy daydreaming feeling of relaxation takes over
Letting go
Drifting down

Deeper and deeper

And your arms, hands, and fingers are relaxing…

Feeling a numb, pleasant, tingling feeling through your fingers as this relaxation grows deeper and deeper.

Neck muscles are relaxing and all the little muscles in the scalp are letting go, feeling as if the blood is circulating very close to the skin.

This relaxation moves down over your forehead and down over your eyelids like a dark veil of sleep as your jaw muscles relax deeply…

Deeply relaxing…

And growing heavier…
And as I count from five to zero, each count will represent deep relaxation and you will feel the body relaxing even more and letting go…

Deeper and deeper…
And when I reach zero, you will go deep asleep.

Now…

Five…letting go

Four…

Three…letting go

Two…

One…

Zero..*(Snap your fingers)*…DEEP ASLEEP!

Now, concentrate on my voice and you will go even deeper asleep with every breath you exhale.

(Time to go to the suggestion you have chosen)

Fall Back Induction

Close your eyes, relax, let go.
You have nowhere to go and nothing to do.
Relax.
I want you to look deep into your imagination
And remember a time in your life that was so wonderful,
So perfect, you wished it would never end
Take a moment to find this time…
Focus on that moment in time
Again, using all the power of your imagination
Now, I want you to safely fall back into that time and place
You can feel your body falling back, relaxed, letting go
Falling back to that moment of bliss
Every muscle in your body, every fiber of your being relaxes
You can hear your self exhale as you reach that state of relief
That state of relaxation
Contentment
Happiness
Relax
Just relax…

(Go to the suggestion of your choice)

Lengthy Induction

Just relax.
Think about what the letters R E L A X mean to you.
Let go.
Relax.

Now take in a deep breath through your nose.
Hold it in while you mentally count to 5.
During this count, gather up all your tensions and frustrations and on the count of 5, strongly exhale them through your mouth.
And relax.
Just relax.

Lets repeat the breathing exercise.

Deep breath in through your nose.
Hold while you count to 5.
Gather up anything that should not be a part of you.
And blow it out through your mouth.

Relax.

Just relax.

Let your breathing become gentle and rhythmic.

Just relax.

Let your body settle gently into your chair, uncross your legs, let the chair support every inch of your physical body.

Relax.

Feel your self sink into the cushions and relax.

Now bring the center of your concentration to your left foot and relax your left foot.
Completely relax your left foot.
Every muscle, tendon, ligament, nerve ending and every molecule.
Completely relax your left foot.

Just relax your left foot.

Now feel the relaxation move up through your ankle, your calf, your knee, your thigh, and into your hip…and relax.

Just relax.

Next, concentrate on you Right foot.
Completely relax your right foot.
Every muscle, tendon, ligament, nerve ending and every molecule.
Completely relax your right foot.

Just relax.

Notice that the entire lower half of your body is now very relaxed and comfortable.
Let it sink into the cushions as you relax.

Now, focus on your lower back.
Your lower back has a tendency to harbor tensions and anxieties.
Let these tensions move out and away from your lower back as you relax.
Relax your lower back.
Deeply.
Completely.
Relax your lower back.

Now, let the relaxation move up your spine.
And as it goes up your vertebrae, it is as if a pair of magical massage hands are kneading each muscle in your back, massaging you, helping you to relax.

And finally the relaxation reaches the back of your neck.
Relax your neck.
Allow the tensions that have found refuge there to move away
And completely relax the back of your neck.
Just relax.

And the relaxation moves up the back of your head, across your scalp, and down over your forehead.
Smoothing out the little worry lines.
Allowing you to relax even deeper.
Relax the little muscles around your eyes.
Just relax.
Part your teeth slightly.
Relax your jaw.
Relax.
Let go.

And the relaxation moves down over your chest, stomach, and abdomen.

Although you are completely relaxed, your organs will continue to function properly, helping you to relax more and more deeply.

Just relax.

Now concentrate on your left shoulder.
Relax your left shoulder.
Every tendon, ligament, nerve ending, and molecule.
Totally relax your left shoulder.
Relax.
Let the relaxation flow down through your upper arm, your elbow, your forearm, your wrist, into your hand, your fingers, and your thumb.
Just relax.
Relax.

Next, concentrate on your right shoulder.
Relax your right shoulder.
Every tendon, ligament, nerve ending, and molecule.
Completely relax your right shoulder.
Relax.
Let the relaxation flow down through your upper arm, your elbow, your forearm, your wrist, into your hand, your fingers, and your thumb.
Just relax.

Let go.

Imagine a wave of relaxation flowing through you from the top of your head to the bottom of your feet.

Just let go.
Just relax.

Now I want you to use the power of your imagination to picture a beautiful downward spiraling staircase in front of you.
Covered is soft thick luxurious carpet.
Winding down with 10 steps.
In a moment, we are going to descend this staircase together.
As we do, I will count backward from 10 to 1 with each descending number taking you deeper down into relaxation.

Let us take our first step down
10
Relax
You can physically feel yourself going down
9
Stepping down, relaxing deeper down

8

Down

Gently down, more deeply relaxed.

7

Just let go and relax as you continue going deeper into relaxation

6

Down, safely, comfortably down

5

Relax

Just relax

4

Deeper relaxed than you have ever been

Going down now to

3

Relax

2

Just completely let yourself relax

1

Where you find yourself more relaxed than you have ever been.

And now you find there is a door in front of you.
Opening the door, you see a beautiful beach outside.
As you step through the door,
You find yourself on a private Caribbean island
On a beautiful day
With the warm sun caressing your skin
And you are so relaxed.
Feel the sand under your feet as you walk along the beach
So safe
So secure
No one to disturb you
On this beautiful day
Somewhere in the Caribbean.
You can feel the gentle breeze against your skin
And taste the salt in the air.
You hear the seagulls in the distance
And you relax
Relax
And as you wander down the beach you find a hammock
Put there just for you.
See yourself gently safely climbing into the hammock
So comfortable
So warm
So safe
So content
And you find yourself rocking gently

Back and forth
Back and forth
So very relaxed
No where to go
Nothing to do but relax
Rocking
Back and forth
Back and forth

There is a trash bag beside the hammock
Pick it up
Begin to reach inside yourself and pull out all things in you that should not be part of
your being
Pull out angers, frustrations, resentments, tensions, and anxieties
What ever is in you that should not be, pull it out and put it in the bag

I am going to be silent for a moment so you can fill your bag
Relax

Now, closing the bag, you can see it magically begin to rise up
The higher it rises, the smaller it appears to be
Until it disappears
Along will all of the garbage that used to be part of you

And you relax
Just relax

(INSERT SUGGESTION)

Relax

Breathing gently and rhythmically

Just relax

In a moment I am going to count from one to five with five being wide awake

When you awaken, you will feel clean, confident, relaxed and ready to take on the world

1
2 beginning to wake up
3 waking up, opening your eyes
4 opening you eyes now
5 wide awake, refreshed, relaxed, and comfortable

Take your time coming back into this moment

Lie there and enjoy the music

You may get up whenever you feel like doing so

SUGGESTIONS

These suggestions are but a few of countless possibilities, limited only by YOUR imagination. Feel free to experiment, keeping your suggestions positive and within the boundaries of your partner's beliefs and ethics. It is NOT unethical to help someone lose his or her inhibitions. Their psyche will provide any necessary limitations.

Hypnotic Suggestions For Performance Enhancement

SPORTS

Are you aware that steroids aren't the only external stimulants used to improve athletic abilities?

The mental side constitutes from 50% to 90% of any given sport. Wayne Gretsky and Tiger Woods are two prevalent examples that come to mind immediately.

Most athletes use Hypnosis in one form or another. Some call it visualization, meditation, or focusing.

Being hypnotized by another seems to be much more effective than self-hypnosis or meditation, as you are guided into your desired mindset and do very little of the effort yourself.

One of my first experiments with hypnosis was with our babysitter. She was running track in high school but performing poorly.

She could never do better than fourth place in the track events.

I invited her over, induced her, and left her with the suggestion that she would feel relaxed and confident at the starting blocks. I further supported this suggestion with a mental image of herself running faster than she had ever run before.

The next day she called to say she had placed first and third in her events!
Since so many of us are now involved in some sort of athletic activity, let's improve our performance and surprise our competition!

I have chosen but a few sports to exemplify. Needless to say, these can be adjusted to suit any sport in which you wish to improve.

Tennis

Continue to relax.

Imagine the atmosphere of the tennis court

Imagine it is a beautiful, sunny day on the court.

Imagine yourself entering into a match.

Even as you remove your racquet cover, you are experiencing a charge of energy while unveiling your weapon.

You grasp the racquet handle and you are immediately confident of the oneness between your arm, your wrist, your hand, and your racquet.

Watching the racquet as you extend your elbow in front of you, you are aware of the strength in each muscle in your arm.

Relaxing your arm for a moment, notice how your legs tighten momentarily, then relax.

Feel the strength, speed, and agility in your legs…and throughout your entire body.

Imagine yourself striding confidently onto the court.

You are alert and your reflexes are well sharpened.

I am going to count from one to five with five being wide awake.

Each and every time you swing your racquet, whether serving or volleying, your entire body will generate a smoothness of motion as you swing through the ball in a confident, professional, and zen-like manner.

Speed, strength, and agility will accompany you throughout each and every game.
1
2
3
4
5…wide awake!

Golf (Driving)

Imagine yourself approaching the Tee.

Striding confidently and relaxed.

Placing the ball, enjoying the fresh air and the feeling of being a fine golfer.

Notice your breathing is in rhythm and harmony with your golf game and will enhance each and every stroke.

Now, picture yourself positioning your body for the drive.

Shoulders, arms, legs…everything exactly as it should be.

There is oneness between the club and you.

Golfing feels very natural to you, as if you had invented it.

Now, imagine yourself bringing the club back, ready to swing.

The weight distribution of the club is absolutely perfect for you.

You can feel its harmony with your skills and enthusiasm.

Your head is still, eyes on the ball.

Picture, in slow motion, the perfect drive.

Swinging through the ball, smoothly…a perfect transition.

Feel the satisfaction tingling every molecule in your body as you so masterfully enjoy this sport.

I am going to count from one to five, with five being wide awake.

Each and every time you approach the Tee on the golf course, you will reflect upon the feeling you have just imagined.

You will be comfortable and confident with your abilities as an outstanding golfer.

1
2
3
4
5…wide awake

Running

Imagine yourself as you begin your morning or evening run. Notice, in slow motion, how your body movements are strong and smooth.

Flowing effortlessly and confidently with each additional stride you take.

Your lungs are clear and healthy. You are a perfect running machine.

Feel the wind you are generating rush by, touching your skin, filling you with even more energy and enthusiasm for running.

Notice that each time your shoes touch down they seem to help you spring into the stride.

In a moment I am going to count from one to five with five being wide awake.

Each and every time you run, your body will feel as though it is the perfect running machine. Your legs and lungs will be filled with the life-force, which creates endurance.

Your movements will be fluid, confident, and comfortable. You will feel as though you are a running machine.

1
2
3
4
5…wide awake!

Sports Recap

These are but a few examples of how to generate performance in sports. As you can tell, we are assisting the body by eliminating undue negative influence from the brain.

Try writing our own script for the sport of your choice. Imagine it as it should be. Concentrate on smoothness of motion, strength, and confidence. Allow for ample visualization.

Be sure your verbiage addresses and overrides any weakness you feel that you may have.

Stage Performance

Whether you are a public speaker, a musician, a singer, or an actor, you are already practicing some form of self-hypnosis to generate confidence each time you step onto the stage.

Do you take a deep breath? Limber up your arms? Tighten your leg muscles and then relax them? Crack your knuckles? These are all forms of mental preparation.

As was pointed out in the sports chapter, being hypnotized by someone else creates a deeper and longer lasting effect.

The following scripts are examples of suggestions that will help your stage performance and confidence levels.

Personally, I suffer from stage fright so this chapter is very dear to my heart.

Guitar

Imagine yourself picking up your guitar. From the beginning, you have known that this is the instrument you love.

Imagine the perfect fit of the contour of the guitar against your torso.

Feel the perfect sizing of the neck as you prepare to play.

Notice the natural way your fingers are able to produce perfection as you touch the strings.

It is as if the frets were arranged just for you.

There is a oneness between you and the guitar.

So natural.

In a moment I am going to count from one to five, with five being wide awake.

Each and every time you play the guitar for someone, you will experience a feeling of confidence in your ability and a oneness with your instrument.

1
2
3
4
5...wide awake!

Public Speaking

Imagine yourself preparing to approach the podium or microphone.

Taking your deep breath in final preparation.

Imagine striding confidently onto the stage. Posture correct. Feeling good.

Your speaking ability is excellent, and you are confident in yourself.

Your throat is clear, your thoughts are organized.

Your breathing is calm and relaxed.

YOU are calm and relaxed.

Throughout the presentation you remain calm, confident and relaxed.

In a moment, I am going to count from one to five with five being wide awake.

Each and every time you make a public speech, you will be calm, confident, and relaxed.

1
2
3
4
5...wide awake!

Singing

Imagine yourself as you are about to sing in front of an audience.

Feeling proud and confident.

Lungs clear. Throat clear.

Feeling enthusiastic. Feeling good!

You have an excellent voice and your audience enjoys your performances.

Focus on your vocal chords and the base of your throat.

Feel the strength and confidence in your physical talent.

Breathing calmly and relaxed.

Feel the strength in your lungs as you sing.

In a moment, I am going to count from one to five with five being wide awake.

Each and every time you sing, you will be confident and relaxed. You will have perfect singing posture. Your throat will remain clear, and your lungs strong.
You will enjoy each moment as it occurs.

1
2
3
4
5…wide awake!

Testing

Recall, concentration, logic, and confidence are the most important psychological factors that affect your performance when taking a test.

There is NO substitute for knowledge!

Again, using hypnosis, we will strengthen these four factors in order to generate improved test scores.

The following hypnotic suggestion should prove quite beneficial the night before your next exam:

Imagine that you are seated at your desk in the classroom awaiting tomorrows _____ exam.

You have prepared yourself thoroughly, eaten properly, and obtained a good nights rest.

You are alert, relaxed and confident in your abilities.

Continue for a few moments to enjoy this feeling of confidence and readiness.

In a moment, I am going to count from one to five with five being wide awake.

Tomorrow, when you enter the examination room and take your seat, you will take a deep breath and relax.

You will reflect for a moment on the feelings you have just imagined.

You will be very alert.

You will find it easy to concentrate on the questions as well as to recall, calculate, or logically deduce the answers. The solutions to each question will come easily and quickly to you.

You will feel relaxed and confident throughout the entire exam.

1
2
3
4
5…wide awake!

Memory

Your ability to remember details, names, data, and other information is consistently improving.

Your memory, your concentration, and your ability to recall information is constantly gaining strength, improving with each passing moment.

You are able to easily retrieve the data stored in you mind.

From this moment forward, you will take pride in your memory skills.

I am going to count from one to five with five being wide awake.
You will feel refreshed and relaxed, more prepared than ever for recollecting the events and information you have stored in your brain.

1
2
3
4
5…wide awake!

Sensual Suggestions

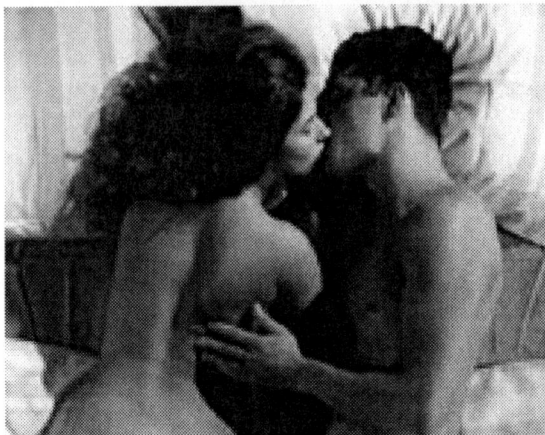

Note:
If your subject is naked while you do this, you
may wish to have a blanket ready for them in the event
they get cold due to slower metabolism.

The Beach

Imagine yourself lying or walking on a white sandy beach.

The sand is white and fine as talcum powder, tinged with pink. The sea is crystal clear, deep turquoise, lapping at your feet.

The breeze is caressing your body and hair.

Feel the warm sun on your body, the sand between your toes, the sea spray on your face.

Now imagine you are lying on the sea, floating.

Feel the buoyancy of the beautiful blue salty water support your body effortlessly as you float on your back, your face upturned toward the sun.

Feel your body become warm as the sun's rays spread their gentle warmth all over you.

Floating. Relaxing.

I am going to count from one to five with five being wide awake.

When you awaken, you will continue to feel warm and relaxed. Oh so comfortable with your self and your body. Proud to be seen in this state of bliss.

1
2
3
4
5…wide awake!

Caribbean Sun

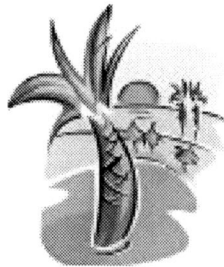

Let your body completely relax.

Imagine the way the warm Caribbean sun feels against your naked tan body.

You are drinking rum punch and it is giving you a very relaxed feeling. Feel the coolness of each sip as it goes down your throat. Feel the increasingly light state of being that accompanies the rum in your body.

You are developing a warm, sensual feeling all over.

Relax. Let go and completely relax.

Let your thinking disappear as your warm body takes complete control of your feelings and actions. Feel free to go with the flow and express yourself openly.

I am going to count from one to five with five being wide awake.

The warm, sensual relaxed feeling will remain with you for the rest of the evening.

1
2
3
4
5…wide awake!

Romantic

Imagine you are in a candle lit room.

You have a glass of wine and the smell of sweet perfume is in the air.

You are feeling very loving and romantic.

You enjoy taking the time to be romantic.

Imagine gentle touches, warm embraces, loving words and looks shared between us.

In a moment, I am going to count from one to five, with five being wide awake.

When you awaken, you will feel even more romantically inclined than you have just imagined.

You will retrieve the wine and insure the candle is lit for us.

The loving, gentle, romantic feeling will remain with you for the remainder of the evening.

1
2
3
4
5…wide awake!

Submission

Relax even deeper. Letting go of all controlling thoughts.

You enjoy being controlled. You do not like to be the one in charge, the one who makes decisions.

You desire to be controlled in every way. You want me to be in complete control tonight.

I may take care of you, your body, and your desires for the rest of the evening.

You have given me complete control.

I am going to count from one to five with five being wide awake.

When you awaken, you will be anxious for me to enjoy you in every possible way.

1
2
3
4
5…wide awake!

Dominance

You enjoy being in control. You are thrilled by the power of absolute domination. You are the boss tonight. The power and control has been awarded to only you.

You have the freedom to do anything you want, any way you wish to do it.

You are in complete control tonight.

Feel the power rising within you now.

I am going to count from one to five, with five being wide awake.

As your eyes open, you will know that the power is within only you.

1
2
3
4
5…wide awake!

Shower

Imagine yourself taking a nice, hot, relaxing shower.

Experience the feel of the lather as you wash your body.

Notice how sensual it feels to wash certain parts of your body.

Feel free to enjoy and explore you entire self in any way you wish for as long as you desire.

Take as much time as you want.

In a moment, I am going to count from one to five, with five being wide awake.

Any time you shower, you will recall the sensual feeling of washing and enjoying your body.

You will treat yourself to ecstasy in the shower by exploring and enjoying all sensual areas of your beautiful body.

1
2
3
4
5…wide awake!

Rum on the Beach

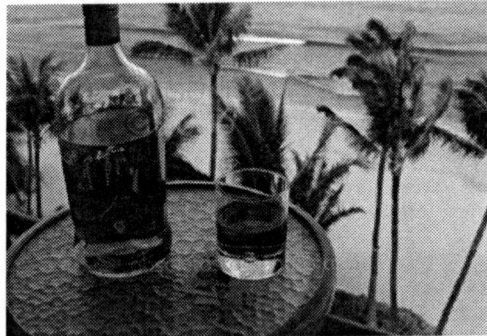

As you continue to relax, imagine the warm white beaches of your favorite tropical environment.

Feel the warmth of the sun on your well-oiled skin.

Your body is feeling relaxed, warm, and comfortable.

Let eh light warm breeze calm you deeper and deeper as it slides across your beautiful skin.

You are so at ease with yourself and the world. Feeling safe, secure, and loved.

Feeling warm and relaxed, imagine taking a large drink of rum.

Feel the alcohol tingle as it enters your body. Let go. Let it work its magic.

Feel the warm tropical sun. So comfortable. You are so happy to be here on this perfect day.

Now, have another sip of your drink. Revel in the way it takes your mind and cares away.

Feel the warmth of the sun on your body.

Everything, every part of you feels so good.

As you continue to drink your potion, you begin to feel a sensation in your private area.

As you have yet another drink, you continue to be more and more stimulated, enjoying the pleasures that come with this feeling.

This feeling is taking away all of your tensions, leaving you feeling very sensual, hot, anxious.

Feel free to have another sip. Continue to release all inhibitions. Who cares? Enjoy!

You have a powerful desire to be touched and make passionate love.

You desire it NOW.

In a moment I am going to count from one to five with five being wide awake.

When you awaken, these feelings will remain with you, very intense, dominating every cavity of your mind.

All you will be able to think about is this warm desirous feeling that has taken over your body and your mind.

You will find exciting ways to satisfy these desires with reckless abandon. Enjoy yourself!

1
2
3
4
5…wide awake!

Sensual Woman

You are a very sensual woman.

Feel your body temperature as it rises a little.

Feel the warmth all over, certain erotic places more so than others.

Enjoy this feeling of warmth as it continues to grow.

Relax as your body becomes more aware of its sexual needs.

Just relax and let yourself feel more and more sensual and erotic.

You cannot stop this feeling.

Allow it to continue to grow.

All the things you thought were important are disappearing. Your feelings of responsibility are no longer relevant. Let go. Enjoy yourself.

The only thing that matters to you is satisfying your sexual needs, urges, and desires.

These desires grow stronger with each passing moment.

They have totally taken control of your body.

Every inch of you is now tingling with desire.

In a moment, I am going to count from one to five with five being wide awake.

When you awaken, your desires and sexuality will dominate your existence for the remainder of the night.

1
2
3
4
5…wide awake!

Naked in the Mountains

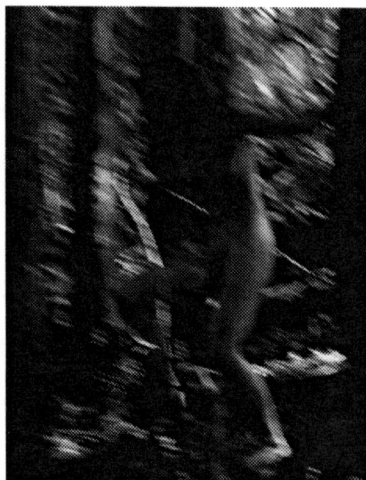

As you continue to relax, imagine yourself transported to a secluded location in the mountains. You have all the privacy in the world. Forest animals are watching but they are quite safe, as are you.

This beautiful spring afternoon has been waiting for you to arrive.

The sun peaks through the branches of the trees. You can hear the rustling of the leaves on the trees and breathe in the fresh mountain air.

Your body longs to be closer to nature. Imagine yourself disrobing. A feeling of freedom immediately drenches your body is happiness.

There you are. Naked on a mountain. No outside influences to disrupt your pleasures. Life is good!

Your partner joins you in nature, disrobing also.

Imagine just the two of you, hidden by the mountain forest, free to express yourselves in any manner you wish.

In a moment I am going to count from one to five with five being wide awake.

When your eyes open, you will continue to feel the freedom and sensual openness of nudity. You will want to play naked with your partner for the remainder of the evening, experiencing all the joys that come with your newfound freedom.

1

2

3

4

5…wide awake!

The following is a complete session on Smoking Cessation leading up to suggestions related to behavior modification. I wish to note at this point, that if someone does not wish to change (i.e. quit smoking) no power on earth can help with the modification.

A Complete Session:
Smoking Cessation

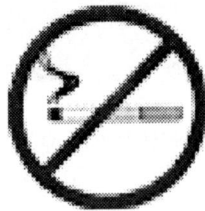

Congratulations!
You have chosen to become a non-smoker and today is the day!

Take a few minutes to insure privacy and quiet for the next hour.
Turn down or off the lights.
Cut off your telephones.
Make sure you will be completely undisturbed.

Make sure you can be totally comfortable.

Now, settle into your chair, relax, and accept that for the next hour or so you have nowhere to go and nothing to do.

For the next hour you will be guided by my voice.
Concentrating only on my voice
Let no outside sounds disturb you
Any sounds you hear will only help you to relax more deeply

Now, Just relax.
Think about what the letters R E L A X mean to you.
Let go.
Relax.

Now take in a deep breath through your nose.
Hold it in while you mentally count to 5.

During this count, gather up all your tensions and frustrations and on the count of 5, strongly exhale them through your mouth.
And relax.
Just relax.

Lets repeat the breathing exercise.

Deep breath in through your nose.
Hold while you count to 5.
Gather up anything that should not be a part of you.
And blow it out through your mouth.

Relax.

Just relax.

Let your breathing become gentle and rhythmic.

Just relax.

Let your body settle gently into your chair, uncross your legs, let the chair support every inch of your physical body.

Relax.

Feel your self sink into the cushions and relax.

Now bring the center of your concentration to your left foot and relax your left foot.
Completely relax your left foot.
Every muscle, tendon, ligament, nerve ending and every molecule.
Completely relax your left foot.

Just relax your left foot.

Now feel the relaxation move up through your ankle, your calf, your knee, your thigh, and into your hip...and relax.

Just relax.

Next, concentrate on you Right foot.
Completely relax your right foot.
Every muscle, tendon, ligament, nerve ending and every molecule.
Completely relax your right foot.

Just relax.

Notice that the entire lower half of your body is now very relaxed and comfortable.
Let it sink into the cushions as you relax.

Now, focus on your lower back.
Your lower back has a tendency to harbor tensions and anxieties.
Let these tensions move out and away from your lower back as you relax.
Relax your lower back.
Deeply.
Completely.
Relax your lower back.

Now, let the relaxation move up your spine.
And as it goes up your vertebrae, it is as if a pair of magical massage hands are kneading each muscle in your back, massaging you, helping you to relax.

And finally the relaxation reaches the back of your neck.
Relax your neck.
Allow the tensions that have found refuge there to move away
And completely relax the back of your neck.
Just relax.

And the relaxation moves up the back of your head, across your scalp, and down over your forehead.
Smoothing out the little worry lines.
Allowing you to relax even deeper.
Relax the little muscles around your eyes.
Just relax.
Part your teeth slightly.
Relax your jaw.
Relax.
Let go.

And the relaxation moves down over your chest, stomach, and abdomen.
Although you are completely relaxed, your organs will continue to function properly, helping you to relax more and more deeply.

Just relax.

Now concentrate on your left shoulder.
Relax your left shoulder.
Every tendon, ligament, nerve ending, and molecule.
Totally relax your left shoulder.
Relax.
Let the relaxation flow down through your upper arm, your elbow, your forearm, your wrist, into your hand, your fingers, and your thumb.
Just relax.

Relax.

Next, concentrate on your right shoulder.
Relax your right shoulder.
Every tendon, ligament, nerve ending, and molecule.
Completely relax your right shoulder.
Relax.
Let the relaxation flow down through your upper arm, your elbow, your forearm, your wrist, into your hand, your fingers, and your thumb.
Just relax.

Let go.

Imagine a wave of relaxation flowing through you from the top of your head to the bottom of your feet.

Just let go.
Just relax.

Now I want you to use the power of your imagination to picture a beautiful downward spiraling staircase in front of you.
Covered is soft thick luxurious carpet.
Winding down with 10 steps.
In a moment, we are going to descend this staircase together.
As we do, I will count backward from 10 to 1 with each descending number taking you deeper down into relaxation.

Let us take our first step down
10
Relax
You can physically feel yourself going down
9
Stepping down, relaxing deeper down
8
Down
Gently down, more deeply relaxed.
7
Just let go and relax as you continue going deeper into relaxation
6
Down, safely, comfortably down
5
Relax
Just relax
4
Deeper relaxed than you have ever been
Going down now to

3
Relax
2
Just completely let yourself relax
1
Where you find yourself more relaxed than you have ever been.

And now you find there is a door in front of you.
Opening the door, you see a beautiful beach outside.
As you step through the door,
You find yourself on a private Caribbean island
On a beautiful day
With the warm sun caressing your skin
And you are so relaxed.
Feel the sand under your feet as you walk along the beach
So safe
So secure
No one to disturb you
On this beautiful day
Somewhere in the Caribbean.
You can feel the gentle breeze against your skin
And taste the salt in the air.
You hear the seagulls in the distance
And you relax
Relax
And as you wander down the beach you find a hammock
Put there just for you.
See yourself gently safely climbing into the hammock
So comfortable
So warm
So safe
So content
And you find yourself rocking gently
Back and forth
Back and forth
So very relaxed
No where to go
Nothing to do but relax
Rocking
Back and forth
Back and forth

There is a trash bag beside the hammock
Pick it up
Begin to reach inside yourself and pull out all things in you that should not be part of
your being

Pull out angers, frustrations, resentments, tensions, and anxieties
What ever is in you that should not be, pull it out and put it in the bag

I am going to be silent for a moment so you can fill your bag
Relax

Now, closing the bag, you can see it magically begin to rise up
The higher it rises, the smaller it appears to be
Until it disappears
Along will all of the garbage that used to be part of you

And you relax
Just relax

As you continue to rock back and forth, breathing gently, so relaxed and comfortable
I want you to see your inner spiritual self, rising safely and comfortably above your
physical self
To a point about 100 feet in the air
As you reach this point, I want you to completely relax and let go

As you look down upon your physical self,
You can see the real you
You can also see the future you

There is a miraculous change about to take place in you
A tingling sensation warms your spirit as you anxiously await these changes

Relax

As you watch, you can see your physical self, transformed into a non-smoker
You can feel closely the problems with the old self as they pass through you
These negatives associated with smoking rise up from your physical body
Pass through your spiritual self
And disappear into space and time
As they leave your physical body, you can sense them approaching
You can smell the odor of smoking as it passes through you and away from you
You can see the blackness it has caused to your lungs as it also passes through you and
away from you
You can taste the breath of smoking as it passes through you and away from you
And see the yellow on your teeth and your skin and your eyes, these too passing through
and leaving your forever

As these feelings pass through you
You rejoice internally
Knowing YOU are a conqueror
A winner

A true champion

You have defeated your worst enemy…The Habit!

Relax

Just relax in your newfound happiness and sense of well-being

Relax

Now, I want you to slowly descend back into your physical body
Gently settling down and in
Like a hand slipping into a glove.

Relax

Breathing gently and rhythmically

Just relax

In a moment I am going to count from one to five with five being wide awake

When you awaken, you will feel clean, confident, relaxed and ready to take on the world
with no escape mechanisms or crutches

You will find that you have no desire for any tobacco products
Not now
Not ever

If your mouth should desire touch, you will be inclined to have a glass of water or Coke

Relax

You are free. You are powerful. You have made a decision to control your life and it
begins NOW

1
2 beginning to wake up
3 waking up, opening your eyes
4 opening you eyes now
5 wide awake, refreshed, relaxed, and comfortable

Take your time coming back into this moment
Lie there and enjoy the music

You may get up whenever you feel like doing so

Additional Behavior Modification Suggestions

Success

Imagine that nothing holds you back from reaching your goal and becoming the successful person that you want to be.

Now, imagine a perfect kind of day. A day that you awaken to and just know it is going to be the kind of day where everything is just right. Everything just falls into place.

You have been comfortable and protected within the boundaries that you yourself have created. You have been comfortable and safe. Now you have chosen to expand your comfort zone.

Just imagine yourself pushing back the barricades your created. Imagine expanding your horizons. Setting and achieving new goals. Thinking outside of the box.

Imagine yourself comfortable with your new goals, boundaries, and horizons.

You feel safe, secure, and pleased that you have the control and power within you to change, to eliminate you previous limitations, and to be the successful person you want to be.

You feel safe, comfortable and at peace.

Now imagine taking this special day and placing it just a little bit in the future. Perhaps a day, a week, or a month. Just a little into the future.

Imagine that you have resolved many conflicts and issues. They are now in the past.

Imagine a smile on your face, you are at peace, content. You have found solutions to problems and you have resolved them.

You are now free of past burdens. You now feel self-assured, centered, and strong. Imagine a goal or project you would like to accomplish.

Place all other minor goals aside and just focus on one goal or project.

See yourself putting energy into your work. See yourself successfully completing it.

You see new opportunities. You see new challenges that are more exciting than the old ones.

See yourself with renewed energy. You are enthusiastic and focused. New ideas develop from the old. New and positive feelings emerge. You are successful.

You reach your goal!

Imagine yourself worthy of all the good things life has to offer.

Reaching your goal is very beneficial to you. As you reach the goals in your life, see them as positive events. Positive for you, your family, friends, and people you work with.

Imagine yourself putting energy into reaching your goals and becoming the successful person you deserve to be.

Reflect for a moment on other positive goals you have already reached.

They were good for you and all those around you.

Now see your self become successful.

You are happy, sensitive to others, helpful, and your success is positive for all.

You are comfortable in your success. You use your success in the most positive and worthwhile ways.

You deserve to be successful. See it. Feel it.

Your mind is clear. You see yourself as the intelligent, creative and beautiful person that you are.

You have many choices, many options. Whatever you choose to do, whatever direction you take, know it will be positive for you.

Your success is a positive event for you and all those who touch your life.

Every choice you make and any path you take is absolutely right for you.

Now just see yourself clearly in the near future. You have many positive directions and choices. Bring this image into the present.

See yourself resolving problems. See yourself confident and successful with many wonderful and positive paths to choose. You know you can continue your success.

You can continue to make choices that enhance your life.

I am going to count from one to five with five being wide awake.

1
2
3
4
5…wide awake!

Weight Control

You feel totally proud of yourself.

You reflect on all the positive things in your life. Recall the goals and successes you have already achieved. Know that you will continue to be successful, reaching every goal that you have set, and creating the most healthy and positive life for yourself.

Now imagine seeing yourself, stomach flat, hips and thighs firm and trim, legs firm and slim. You look great and feel so good!

You are relaxed and peaceful. Food is less and less important. You are more comfortable eating more slowly.

Snacking is unimportant to you, regardless of where you are or what you're doing. You can eat small amounts of food in a restaurant and you will eat more slowly.

You may leave part of your meal on your plate, and that is fine.

Regardless of stress, you are more at peace and relaxed. Food is less important to you. You feel proud of yourself.

The rewards are tremendous.

And now, whenever you think of eating, you choose those good healthful foods. You choose to eat the correct amount.

When you have eaten the correct amount, you stop eating. You simply stop eating.

You may even leave some food on your plate and that is just fine. You simply stop eating.

Continue to relax. Allow that sense of confidence and peace to flow through you now.

You are motivated now more than ever before to create the most healthy and positive life for yourself. You are motivated to change old eating patterns into good eating patterns. You are motivated to lose the amount of weight you no longer want or need. You are compelled to maintain this weight loss.

I am going to count from one to five with five being wide awake.

1
2
3
4
5…wide awake!

Stress Management

Because you are now relaxed, let any feelings you have buried come up to the surface.

Examine these feelings.

Decide which ones you want to keep and which ones you want to discard. Keep the ones you need right now, and cast away the others.

It is all right for you to feel sad or depressed sometimes. It is your way of being good to yourself. Depression is a healing process. You can allow yourself to mourn or be sad. When you have completed the time of sadness, set yourself free.

You are good to yourself and the time will soon be over for those feelings. You will feel free from them because you will be able to accept or discard any feelings at all.

Discard any feelings you are through with. They are yours and you can let them come and go as you need them.

Now, relax, and continue to relax. Feel yourself relaxed with your feelings.

Think of how you are a whole person with many feeling that make you whole and healthy. If unwanted outside pressure comes at you, you are surrounded by a shield that protects you from pressure.

The shield will protect you from pressures invading you.
Pressure bounces off and away from you. No matter where it comes from or who sends it, it just bounces off and away.

You feel fine because the shield protects you all day from stress and pressure. You go through your day feeling just fine.

You watch the stress bounce off and away. The more stress outside, the calmer you feel inside.

You feel calm inside.

You are a calm person and you are shielded from stress.

You act in ways that make you feel good. Your days will be full of accomplishments which will please you.

You are calm and strong. Free from Stress. Totally free from Stress.

I am going to count from one to five, with five being wide awake.

1
2
3
4
5…wide awake!

Concentration

Concentrate on one side of your brain and one eye.

Imagine with your right eye, and with the right side of your brain, that you see a tree in spring covered with pink and white blossoms.

Now, using the left side of your brain, and then the left eye, see the same tree draped in snow.

Establish these two pictures clearly and distinctly.

Now try to merge the images of the two trees into the center of your brain where they become one tree covered in autumn foliage.

Relax and enjoy the image you have created.

Your concentration skills are improving. The more you practice such techniques, the more honed they will become.

In a moment, I am going to count from one to five with five being wide awake.

When you awaken, you will be able to concentrate with both sides of your brain as well as with the center of your brain.

1
2
3
4
5…wide awake!

The following is a course unto itself. It contains a complete explanation, induction, suggestion, and release that can change your world. Take it seriously when you do it and wonderful things will happen.

A Complete session:

Superbolic Metabolism
(Healing Via Cell Memory

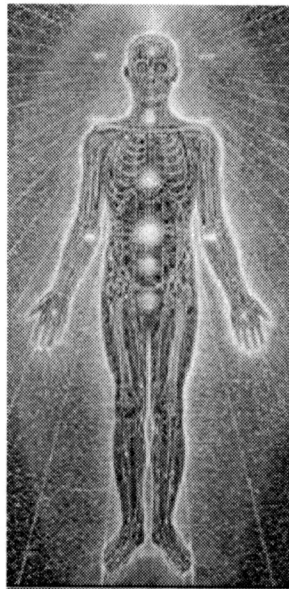

The overall purpose of this journey is to resurrect the healing power within each of us, or as the Army says: To Be All That You Can Be.

Let us begin with our breathing.
Take a deep breath in through your nose,
Holding it in whiling you mentally count to five.
While counting, gather up all of your tensions, anxieties, fears, and frustrations
Then, on the count of five, strongly exhale them through your mouth
Releasing all of these feelings and emotions
Let go
And relax.

Let's try it again.
Take a deep breath in through your nose,
Holding it in while mentally counting to five.
During the count, gather up all frustrations and tensions that have no business being in you
Then, on the count of 5
Vehemently exhale, blowing out all of these emotions
And relax
Just relax

Allow your breathing to become gentle and rhythmic as you just let go and relax.

Now, here are the fundamentals.

Your brain sends signals to each cell in your body.
Any and all signals will be reacted to accordingly, as well as memorized by each of your cells.

Let me show you an example of this signal versus reaction theory:
Close your eyes, relax, and let go for a moment.
Imagine that in front of you is a big ripe yellow juicy lemon.
Now, see yourself slicing the lemon in half.
Next, slice one of the halves in half.
Imagine picking it up.
Now, take a bite of it.
Did your mouth respond?
Was there really a lemon there to cause such response?

Knowing what you know now, does it not make sense that if you experience stress, your brain will not only create a reaction in you, it will also develop a detrimental memory in each of your cells so that future events will be interpreted and reacted to in a like manner.

Our cells, all the millions of them, are each quite miraculous.
They are designed to regenerate themselves perpetually.
This is called anabolic metabolism.
Unfortunately, our reactions to negative perceptions, stress, pain, and so forth, cause this regenerative process to be interrupted or to cease.
This negative cell action is referred to as catabolic metabolism.

Man did not experience these effects until the industrial age and
the subsequent evolution of society into modern day man.
The decisions that made fighting unacceptable as a means to resolve issues and the pursuit of the almighty dollar have lead us to where we are today.
As a result of these changes in society, we now experience
Faster heart rates, higher blood pressure, anxiety, apprehension, and a fear of the unknown.

This is not to mention the extent to which our health degenerates with the influx of these stressors.

Pressure builds up inside. We overcompensate. Eventually we loose the will to fight and end up depressed and apathetic.

This catabolic process is what causes us to age, develop cancer, clog arteries, and so forth, and so on.

Can you imagine altering the flow of data from the brain to the cells in a manner that would deter aging and block cancer?

We call this process SuperBolic© Metabolism, the modification of non-recent cell memory at a sub-conscious level, as an alleviation of catabolic metabolism.
The terminology here is not the important part so if you find it confusing, just let it go and get on with the program.

Here is the important part:
What you put into this program and the level in which you accept it will be directly proportionate to the results you achieve from it.

You will be guided into a heightened state of relaxation during the next hour.
You may find that your conscious mind will remain active all the while.
This is not unusual.
Most communication from me will be dealing with subconscious levels of acceptance and can in no way harm you.
Contrary to some stories, you will not do, think, or feel anything that is against your personal beliefs.
The worst effect possible is that you will have the equivalent of 2 to 4 hours rest during this time.

You are in control at all times and if you wish to stop for any reason, you have only to open your eyes and cease participation.

There are three things you MUST do to supplement this program.
Practice, practice, practice.

As this will be an entirely unique concept to your brain, it may need time to become acclimated in order to achieve the desired results.

Now, let's get started.

Take a few moments to adjust yourself in your recliner.
Make certain that each part of your physical body is supported fully so that you may totally relax.

The more comfortable you are, the more effective you will find this program to be.

Again, for the next hour, you have nowhere to go and nothing to do.

Now, just relax.
Completely relax.
Your day is behind you, along with all of its' tensions and stressors.
There is only this moment in time.
Any events that happened before this moment, as well as any events that may occur later, are irrelevant and have no bearing on this moment.
You are here and now.
Nothing more.
You are safe and comfortable.
Nothing else matters for the next hour.
Just relax.

Think about what the letters R E L A X mean to you.

Just let go.
Just Relax.

Now take in a deep breath through your nose.
Hold it in while you mentally count to 5.
During this count, gather up all your tensions and frustrations and on the count of 5, strongly exhale them through your mouth.
And relax.
Just relax.

Lets repeat the breathing exercise.

Deep breath in through your nose.
Hold while you count to 5.
Gather up anything that should not be a part of you.
And blow it out through your mouth.

Relax.

Just relax.

Let your breathing become gentle and rhythmic.

Just relax.

Let your body settle gently into your chair, uncross your legs, let the chair support every inch of your physical body.

Relax.

Feel your self sink into the cushions and relax.

Now bring the center of your concentration to your left foot and relax your left foot.
Completely relax your left foot.
Every muscle, tendon, ligament, nerve ending and every molecule.
Completely relax your left foot.

Just relax your left foot.

Now feel the relaxation move up through your ankle, your calf, your knee, your thigh, and into your hip…and relax.

Just relax.

Next, concentrate on you Right foot.
Completely relax your right foot.
Every muscle, tendon, ligament, nerve ending and every molecule.
Completely relax your right foot.

Just relax.

Notice that the entire lower half of your body is now very relaxed and comfortable.
Let it sink into the cushions as you relax.

Now, focus on your lower back.
Your lower back has a tendency to harbor tensions and anxieties.
Let these tensions move out and away from your lower back as you relax.
Relax your lower back.
Deeply.
Completely.
Relax your lower back.

Now, let the relaxation move up your spine.
And as it goes up your vertebrae, it is as if a pair of magical massage hands are kneading each muscle in your back, massaging you, helping you to relax.

And finally the relaxation reaches the back of your neck.
Relax your neck.
Allow the tensions that have found refuge there to move away
And completely relax the back of your neck.
Just relax.

And the relaxation moves up the back of your head, across your scalp, and down over your forehead.

Smoothing out the little worry lines.
Allowing you to relax even deeper.
Relax the little muscles around your eyes.
Just relax.
Part your teeth slightly.
Relax your jaw.
Relax.
Let go.

And the relaxation moves down over your chest, stomach, and abdomen.
Although you are completely relaxed, your organs will continue to function properly, helping you to relax more and more deeply.

Just relax.

Now concentrate on your left shoulder.
Relax your left shoulder.
Every tendon, ligament, nerve ending, and molecule.
Totally relax your left shoulder.
Relax.
Let the relaxation flow down through your upper arm, your elbow, your forearm, your wrist, into your hand, your fingers, and your thumb.
Just relax.
Relax.

Next, concentrate on your right shoulder.
Relax your right shoulder.
Every tendon, ligament, nerve ending, and molecule.
Completely relax your right shoulder.
Relax.
Let the relaxation flow down through your upper arm, your elbow, your forearm, your wrist, into your hand, your fingers, and your thumb.
Just relax.

Let go.

Imagine a wave of relaxation flowing through you from the top of your head to the bottom of your feet.

Just let go.
Just relax.

Now I want you to use the power of your imagination to picture a beautiful downward spiraling staircase in front of you.
Covered is soft thick luxurious carpet.
Winding down with 10 steps.

In a moment, we are going to descend this staircase together.
As we do, I will count backward from 10 to 1 with each descending number taking you deeper down into relaxation.

Let us take our first step down
10
Relax
You can physically feel yourself going down
9
Stepping down, relaxing deeper down
8
Down
Gently down, more deeply relaxed.
7
Just let go and relax as you continue going deeper into relaxation
6
Down, safely, comfortably down
5
Relax
Just relax
4
Deeper relaxed than you have ever been
Going down now to
3
Relax
2
Just completely let yourself relax
1
Where you find yourself more relaxed than you have ever been.

And now you find there is a door in front of you.
Opening the door, you see a beautiful beach outside.
As you step through the door,
You find yourself on a private Caribbean island
On a beautiful day
With the warm sun caressing your skin
And you are so relaxed.
Feel the sand under your feet as you walk along the beach
So safe
So secure
No one to disturb you
On this beautiful day
Somewhere in the Caribbean.
You can feel the gentle breeze against your skin
And taste the salt in the air.
You hear the seagulls in the distance

And you relax
Relax
And as you wander down the beach you find a hammock
Put there just for you.
See yourself gently safely climbing into the hammock
So comfortable
So warm
So safe
So content
And you find yourself rocking gently
Back and forth
Back and forth
So very relaxed
No where to go
Nothing to do but relax
Rocking
Back and forth
Back and forth

There is a trash bag beside the hammock
Pick it up
Begin to reach inside yourself and pull out all things in you that should not be part of
your being
Pull out angers, frustrations, resentments, tensions, and anxieties
What ever is in you that should not be, pull it out and put it in the bag

I am going to be silent for a moment so you can fill your bag
Relax

Now, closing the bag, you can see it magically begin to rise up
The higher it rises, the smaller it appears to be
Until it disappears
Along will all of the garbage that used to be part of you

And you relax
Just relax

Now, as you continue to rock back and forth in your hammock,
free from the burdens you previously carried unnecessarily,
enjoying each sensation,
the sun, the breeze, the taste of salt air, the sound of seagulls,
Know that all is well and that the powers of the universe, the energy of existence, and
God as you know him are all gathered in you and around you at this moment in time to
re-give you the strength, power, and wisdom to live a healthy, perfect life.

I want you to pay close attention to the life force within you, the God force residing in your abdomen and in your heart.
Take a moment to feel the power within you.

Now notice that there is a tingling in each cell in your body, from the top of your head to the bottom of your feet
The tingling sensations are your cells, all acknowledging that they are listening.
Take a moment to experience this incredible feeling.

As you continue to experience the presence of your life force and the tingling of each cell in your body, accept that your physical body is about to undergo a phenomenal change.

Because of the profound nature of the mind-body experience, you may come to tears and this is absolutely okay. Do not be afraid to let the tears flow.

This is a moment of great joy and you are free to feel the joy to the depths of your being.

Now, using the power of your imagination, I want you to allow your spiritual self to rise up in the air to a point about 100 feet above the ground.

Relax.

From this point you may witness the miracles that are about to occur in your physical being.

In a moment I am going to count backwards from 3 to one.
At the count of one, your cells and thusly your physical body will not longer be willing or able to accept any stress signals, either new or existing from your subconscious mind.
Any information that was previously stored in your cells which was less than healthy, loving, and good will be removed.

Your subconscious mind can and will, from this moment forward, store all stress related information in compartments in the back of your brain. These stressful events and occurrences may be retained for information only. They no longer affect you at any level of life except when used to make healthy choices for yourself.

Your active front part of your brain will find peace and happiness in every moment of life, acknowledging the storage of all damaging information in a safe place where it can in no way bring harm or discomfort to you.

Now, as I countdown, each cell in your body will become cleansed and healthy.
Three
Two
One.
Each cell is now allowed and expected to repair and regenerate itself as it was originally designed to do.

Information of a negative or stressful nature may no longer enter into your cells.
It will from this moment on be compartmentalized safely in the back of your mind for information purposes only.

You can already feel the changes within you. This feeling will remain with you at all times as a reminder of your freedom from stress, disease, and aging.

Now, I want you to descend back down to earth. Back down into your physical being.
Slowly, gently re-entering your body.
Like a hand sliding into a glove.
Comfortable and relaxed.

Feeling the new life within each cell of your being.

In a moment, I am going to count from 1 to 5, with 5 being wide awake.
When you awaken, you will feel the power within you and the tingling from head to toe which indicates your success in accepting the healthy healing power which you have chosen to be a permanent part of your being.

Always remember, you made this choice, and it is good.

1
2   waking up
3   opening your eyes
4   waking up
5   now wide awake, refreshed, cleansed, healthy, and relaxed

Congratulations

Enjoy each moment that life brings you from this moment on……..

Take several moments to regain your composure. There is no rush to get up.

Just For Fun

Laughter therapy

Recall a funny incident, a comedy movie, a joke you heard.

Think about it and let yourself laugh, feeling the corners of your mouth turn up, letting your self laugh…a hearty laugh.

Feel it vibrate through your body.

When you finish laughing, experience a sense of release and well-being and keep that feeling of well-being with you throughout the day.

I am going to count from one to five with five being wide awake

1
2
3
4
5…wide awake!

Energy

In a moment I am going to count from one to five with five being wide awake.

When you awaken you will be full of energy and enthusiasm, yet calm and relaxed on the inside. No one can take away your inner feeling of relaxation.

1
2
3
4
5…wide awake!

Sleeping Arm

In a moment, I am going to count from one to five with five being wide awake.

When you awaken, you will find that your left arm has become numb. Your left arm has gone completely to sleep and you cannot wake it up.

The harder you try to get your left arm to function, the more deeply it goes to sleep.

1
2
3
4
5…wide awake!

X-Ray Vision

In a moment, I am going to count from one to five with five being wide awake.

When you awaken you will find that you have the same X-Ray vision as Superman.

You are now able to see through other peoples clothing. You can see everything underneath other peoples clothing.

You are comfortable seeing through peoples clothes.

1
2
3
4
5…wide awake!

(Watch the expression on their face!)

French

In a moment, I am going to count from one to five with five being wide awake.

When you awaken, you will find that you speak only French. You have acquired a thorough understanding of French. You speak no English. You understand no English. Only French.

You are very comfortable speaking only French.

1
2
3
4
5…wide awake!

(This one turned ME into a cocky Parisian. I must admit it was FUN!)

Smiling

In a moment, I am going to count from one to five with five being wide awake.

When you awaken you will be smiling and happy. Everything is right with your world and everything is good.

Everyone loves you and you love everyone.

Your eyes sparkle and you want to show everyone how much you love him or her.

You feel healthy, vibrant, and full of life.

1
2
3
4
5…wide awake!

Elvis

In a moment, I am going to count from one to five with five being wide awake.

When you awaken, you will be the world's greatest Elvis impersonator and you will perform your favorite Elvis song as if you were on stage.

You feel very comfortable being such a great Elvis impersonator.

1
2
3
4
5...wide awake!

Shoes

In a moment, I am going to count from one to five with five being wide awake.

You will notice that your shoes are on the wrong feet. You will immediately put them on the other foot.

1
2
3
4
5…wide awake!

Telephone

In a moment, I am going to count from one to five with five being wide awake.

Each and every time you hear a telephone ring, you will yell out "Who the Hell Is It?" And then answer the phone in a calm and normal manner.

1
2
3
4
5…wide awake!

Forget Your Name

In a moment I am going to count from one to five with five being wide awake.

When you awaken you will be unable to remember anyone's name. You cannot even remember your own name. You know where you are but you cannot remember your name or anyone else's.

1
2
3
4
5...wide awake!

He Becomes She

Inside each of us is both male and female.

The female part of you is taking control and you like it.

You are feeling very feminine all over.
Notice the way you now want to hold your legs, your hands.
Feel your posture changing.
Can you feel the difference in you eyes?
Your lips?
Do you need lipstick?
You can even feel changes in your hair.

You feel like a woman.
You are a sexy woman.
You ARE a woman.

I am going to count from one to five with five being wide awake.

When you awaken, every part of you will be that of a woman.

1
2
3
4
5...wide awake!

(Without going into detail, I will say I was amazed at the results of this one)

Wine

In a moment, I am going to count from one to five with five being wide awake.

When you awaken, each and every sip of wine or water you take will affect you as if you had consumed an entire BOTTLE of wine.

The third sip will render you speechless and unable to focus your eyes clearly.

Relax and enjoy this oncoming state of inebriation.

When I snap my fingers you will become immediately sober

1
2
3
4
5…wide awake!

The next two regression sessions are not to be taken lightly. Please pay close attention to what you are doing and to how your subject is responding.

Age Regression Script (After Induction)

You can take a deep breath, and you will note that a drifting can occur – that there is less and less importance to be attached to my voice.

In due time, your own time, a minute, an hour, a week, a month, some time, your subconscious will reveal its gifts to you in a dream or in a daydream when you're not especially thinking about it. Memories of other times and other places. Memories you only thought you had misplaced. Experiences you only thought you had mislaid.

With this new insight, comes new growth and new understanding.

Stored deep in your subconscious are wonderful memories.

Your subconscious can call upon and access these memories and bring them back with you later.

So, by looking deeper into the recesses of your own mind you can see your soul's vision and hear the voice of your heart.

Later, you can apply this knowledge to better understand yourself and your world.

In a moment, we can begin a series of exercise into memory, perception, and recall.

Can you remember a time in your life when you really felt safe and comfortable?

You may begin now going back to about the time you were 18 years old. Choosing a pleasant, happy memory of about the time that you were 18 years old.

You will find that it is very easy for you to do this... choosing one specific memory or one specific event... and just simply focusing on it. Look at the people around you. Now look at yourself.

I will be quiet and give you ample time to simply enjoy this event.

You may hear voices, you ay see or feel the people.

It may be in vivid color, as in a cinema movie.

The images may be black and white or just vague outlines.

You may hear the memory.

Sometimes a certain smell will trigger the memory.

You are about 18 years old now. What is happening?

(The hypnotist needs to be VERY patient during this part)

Now, you may continue back, going back now to about the time that you were five years old.

Again, choosing a pleasant, happy memory, an impression, an episode, any memory you wish.

Look at it clearly.

See what you were wearing. Sense or feel the people around you.

Look and listen to the information. Reach down deep and feel it, and I will be quiet.

In a moment, I am going to count from one to five with five being wide awake. When you awaken, you will be five years old.

You will be happy, feeling young.

(patiently enjoy your partner as a five year old)

When I snap my fingers, you will return to the deep state of relaxation. You will sleep.

Now your journey is concluded.

Once again I am going to count from one to five with five being wide awake. You will awaken to find yourself back in the present.

You will be able to recall critically and analytically all that you have just experienced.

1
2
3
4
5…wide awake!

Past Life Regression

Please read this very carefully before embarking on your adventure

Introduction:

Past life regression, supposedly, is a hypnotic method of viewing your past lives, assuming the validity of reincarnation theory.

I assume and suppose because there is no way to prove what you experience during this exciting voyage.

The source of all the data which will be revealed is arguable, so feel free to choose your own opinion. Either way, it is unforgettable.

Should you choose to continue this adventure, allow yourself a couple of hours for the session and the conversation which will follow.

Trust me on this one…a very serious attentive attitude is mandatory!

You will be tempted to laugh or gasp or react in some manner…YOU CAN NOT DO IT!

Noises of this nature will snap your subject out of the trance and wipe out all of your hard work. Do it with diligence or do not bother.

This is guaranteed to be far more interesting than any sit-com on Television and much healthier for you than CNN.

(Induction:)

Take a deep breath and relax.

Move to the center of your consciousness, the very center, to the muscles of your eyelids.

Become aware that all the tension is pouring right out and you are relaxing.

Relax. Just relax.

Now become aware of your eyes. Just let your eyes relax. Feel them relaxing and releasing.

Relax.
Relax.

Now move the center of your awareness down to the muscles of the upper part of your face. Become aware of them. Relax.

Just Relax
Relax

Now become aware of your cheeks. Feel all the tension just drain out of your cheeks.

Relax
Relax
Relax

Now become aware of the muscles around your mouth. And your lips. Just feel all the tension come out. And relax.

Relax
Relax

Feel the muscles of your jaw become loose. You just feel those muscles relax. The jaw drops down from its relaxation.

Relax
Relax

You will find that if you need to swallow, you can do so naturally and still remain very, very relaxed.

Now, feel the muscles of your forehead. Become aware of those muscles. Feel them relax.

Relax
Relax

Now, in total relaxation, move back across the muscles of your scalp. Feel the muscles of your scalp relax.

Relax
Relax

Now move the center of your awareness back to the muscles of the back of the head, the back of your neck, and relax.

Relax
Just relax

Your whole head is feeling so relaxed. You become aware of how heavy it feels. It feels so relaxed, so heavy, that it is just weighing down into the cushion.

Bring the center of your awareness to your nostrils. Become aware of your nostrils. Become aware of your nostrils. Feel the air going back and forth.

Back and forth
Relax
Back and forth
Relax

Feel how good it feels to have air going through your nostrils into your nose…right down your throat and into your lungs.

Feel the wonderful movement through your lungs as it moves in and out.

Feel how the free flow of air makes you feel more and more relaxed. More and more comfortable. Deeper and deeper into relaxation.

Now feel as you take a deep breath, as deep as you can, feel the muscles of your chest wall relax.

More and more relaxed.

Feel the relaxation going down to the muscles of the abdomen. Become aware of those muscles.

Relax
Relax

You are very very relaxed.

Now become aware of the muscles from the base of your neck, to the base of your spine.

Pay close attention to all the muscles of your spine.

Relax
Relax
Relax

Now feel the upper part of your body slowly relax. Feel the weight of it as it slowly unwinds.

It is feeling heavy.

It is feeling very, very heavy.

Now begin to relax your shoulders. Your right shoulder. Focus all you attention to that shoulder and let it relax.

Relax
Relax

Now feel the muscles of your right arm relax. Feel those muscles relax.

Relax
Relax

Now move the center of your awareness down into the muscles of your right forearm. Become aware of those muscles. Let them relax.

Relax
Relax

Now move your awareness to the muscles of your right wrist and hand. All around to the tips of your fingers. Just let them relax.

Relax
Relax

Now move the center of your awareness to your left shoulder. Focus all of your attention to that shoulder and let it relax.

Relax
Relax
Relax

Now feel the muscles of your left arm relax, Feel those muscles relax.

Relax
Relax

Now move the center of your awareness down into the muscles of your left forearm. Become aware of those muscles. Let them relax.

Relax
Relax
Relax

Now move your awareness to the muscles of your left wrist and hand. All around to the tips of your fingers. Just let them relax.

Relax
Relax

Now bring the center of your consciousness over to the muscles of your left leg. Now feel your left upper thigh begin to relax. Feel this relaxation going down to your knee. Become aware of those muscles and relax.

Relax
Relax
Relax

Now feel the relaxation going down to your left lower leg. Down through your calf. All the way out through the tips from your toes. Now relax.

Just relax
Relax
Notice that your whole left side, from the top of your head to the tips of your toes feels so heavy, so relaxed.

YOU feel very, very relaxed.

Your whole body is feeling so heavy. It just feels as though it is sinking down into the cushions.

And if you feel as though your mouth is dry, you can help that by moving your consciousness right down to the pit of your stomach.

Now I am going to count down, from ten to zero. With each count downward, you are going to be more and more deeply relaxed.

Until the count of zero, you will be a deeply relaxed and comfortable as you can be at this moment in time.

Now bring the center of your consciousness over to the muscles of your right leg. Now feel your right upper thigh begin to relax. Feel this relaxation going down to you knee. Become aware of those muscles and relax.

Relax
Relax
Relax

Now feel the relaxation going down to your right lower leg. Down through your calf. All the way out through the tips of your toes. Now relax

Just let go and relax
Relax

Relax

Notice that your whole right side, from the top of your head to the tips of your toes, feels so heavy. So relaxed.

And with each count downward you will feel more and more relaxed. Very, very comfortable.

Ten. You are feeling ore deeply relaxed.

Nine. You are deeper, deeper, and deeper. You are more comfortable and relaxed.

Eight. You are deeper, deeper, deeper down. All the way to…

Seven. Deeper, deeper, becoming more and more comfortable. Down to …

Six. Deeper down. Deeper down.

Five. You are feeling more and more deeply relaxed all the way to…

Four. Deeper and deeper. More relaxed.

Three. Going deeper down now into relaxation. Down to…

Two. Deeper down.

One. Now deeper down than ever before. You are very relaxed.

Zero. Here you are more deeply relaxed and comfortable than you have ever been.

Now I want you to stay very relaxed and comfortable.

I want you to imagine that you are in a beautiful place. It is a wonderful, safe, comfortable place. Use the power of your mind to imagine this beautiful spot outdoors.

Look all around you and see your surroundings vividly. Picture how it looks and feel the comfort that you have in this place.

(PLR Suggestion)

In a moment I am going to ask you to uses the power of your mind and imagination.

To imagine, to feel that you rise upward out of your body on this beautiful day. To a point of view several hundred feet above yourself.

From that point, you will descend gradually until you come back down to earth again. But this time, when your feet hit the ground, you will find yourself in a previous life. In an experience that feels very much like a life you have led sometime in the past. Before you were born.

You will be able to go in and out of them.

Even though you are very deeply relaxed, you will be able to talk and simultaneously the feelings, thoughts, and scenes will come to mind.
And, if you wish, you will be able to disengage your critical faculties and just let whatever comes up to your mind surface.

You will be able to go with it.

Later on, you will be able to look back on it critically and analytically if you wish. But for now, just let it happen.

The experience will come. And you will find that throughout this experience your body will be relaxed and comfortable.

You may experience the emotions that come along with any events. If you do, you will feel completely confident that these emotions can in no way harm you now.

You have lived through them before and you know that you are safe.

Now, from this beautiful spot, feel the life-force within you, that tingling energy in your body.

Feel yourself rising up above your body. Use the power of the mind to picture it. There you are. You are feeling so comfortable. So relaxed.

In a moment, I will snap my fingers and your unconscious mind will select a past life which is particularly relevant and interesting to your life now.

Just relax and let your subconscious mind to the work. Let it select the life.

S N A P

Now, feel yourself drift slowly down. Down. Down. Now slowly, gently, ready to touch the ground.

Remember that when you touch the ground you will remember a past and you will accept what you see.

You are drifting down, slowly settling down to the ground. You are looking down at your feet.

Can you see your feet?

(Always patiently wait for the subject to respond and pay very close attention to their actions.)

Look at the ground around your feet.

Now slowly look up.

Slowly.

Be willing to accept what you see.

Slowly look up. Be willing to accept what you see.

You should be looking straight ahead now.

The world around you should be coming slowly into focus.
Slowly into focus.

Things should be clearer now.

Clearer

Focus now and accept what you see.

Accept your surroundings.

Now, when I count three, tell me what you see.

One…

Two…

Three…

Now tell me what you see in this past life.

(Listen patiently)

Tell me more.

If you can tell me more, please do. But do not feel pressured. Tell me what you see, if anything.

Are there any people?

If you see any, what are they wearing and what do they look like?

What does the surrounding area look like?

Talk about what you see. Are there buildings or structures of any kind?

What is the geography like?

Tell me.

Tell me more about the surroundings in this past life if you can.

Feel free to move around in this past life.

Explore at will. Examine things around you. Look at this past life with wonder. Tell me what you see.

Can you hear any conversations?

Do you know your name?

How old are you?

Do you have family?

Describe what you see and hear. I am listening.

Do you hear conversations now?

Do you see anyone in this past life who is with you in your present life?

If you do, tell me about them. Who are they and how are they treating you?

You can move through time in this past life. Move to the end of this life and tell me what you see.

How do you look?

Where are you? Describe your surroundings.

I want you to tell me what is happening at this point in your past life. I will be silent for a couple of minutes while you describe in all the detail you can what is happening. Go ahead and talk.

Okay. Is there more?

Okay. Freeze this past life where it is.

You are in control of these events so you can certainly do what you wish.

I want you to remember that this was a past life. You are in another life now and whatever happened in that past life was something you lived through. You can learn to live better and more happily in your current life through the experiences in your past life.

You are going to come gently back to your current life. Feel yourself drift slowly down into your body. Slowly. Slowly.

Feel your subconscious letting go of the past life and returning to your body.

Slowly. Gently. It is slipping back inside of you like a hand in a glove.

Can you feel it? You are back inside of your body.

Gently move your hands and feet.

Gently move your head from side to side.

Take three deep breaths.

One…

Two…

Three…

You are back now. Open your eyes and become aware of your surroundings. I am finished now, but you should lie there a few minutes more and think about the past life you just experienced. Does it relate to your present life? Are there lessons that can be learned from it?

Now, wide awake and feeling good.

Some Past Life Experiences

Quoted experiences from some clients:

" My first experience with Past Life Regression took me back in time via automobile. When I first arrived it was dark and I thought I must be a cave woman or something from prehistoric times. Everything was dark and I was alone.

Next I was instructed to remember the most dramatic happening of this lifetime and I envisioned a white house, with a person in a long white robe, sitting on this horse. Everything was very bright and white.

Next I was instructed to see the person who caused me the most anxiety in this life. I saw a woman with short to medium pageboy hair (black) who was aged and scowling at me. I was also asked my name which came immediately: DICA.

Finally I was asked to envision my death. I saw a man with an animal head (wolf perhaps) chanting and shaking noise over my body near on open fire. I lay there stretched out in white with long dark hair and I appeared to be old.

This was when I realized that I might be a cave dwelling Indian and perhaps this was my burial by a medicine man.

In this life I was never married and had no children"

" I arrived as Karen. I was surrounded by my children on the prairie. We had beautiful church clothes on. I was in a print long dress with light longer hair. About four children were around me, all girls with bonnets.

I pictured my little house on the prairie. Inside, I was sewing and cooking. My husband sat at a desk with a lantern on and our gazes met as we smiled. We were very happy.

This session seemed to end to soon as I was brought back to reality."

" The lifting up of my body before coming down to earth was a little scary, as I found my self physically rising above the bed.

I could feel the top of my loose jeans against my legs. When I came down to earth and saw myself, What a surprise!

My shoes were black with designer holes around the tops. I knew I was a man!

I saw my house, a beautiful big country mansion. One side of the road to the house had big trees lining the road. All colors were autumn and the leaves rustled around me.

Next I was in my house, perhaps in the study. I had a leather chair. I was handsome, around 35040 years old. Sandy hair, physically fit, wearing a paisley smoking jacket and smoking a pipe. My name was Kevin MacGregor.

There was a cocker spaniel that jumped on my lap and I had a fire burning in the fireplace next to my chair. A large window viewed my front yard. The foyer was off to my left.

As I was looking out the window, I noticed a familiar woman with two boys coming to my door. I met them in the foyer. The younger boy, maybe 4, clung closely to his mother. I was then asked their names. Betty was the woman and she was either my sister or sister-in-law.

The older boy was named John and he was standing very tall next to his mother. He wore a brown coat and knickers. He had short reddish hair and his ears stuck out.
I forget the younger boys name.
My death scene showed me as older with white hair and a long full curly beard. I was dressed in dark clothing and a top hat. As I stepped out onto a cobblestone road from a door in town, I was struck by the wheel of a carriage (large wheel).
They could not see me. It was dark and I was dressed so dark. That was how this life ended."

One of my own experiences:

"I landed as a Norse barmaid, Nikki! Quite clearly I was standing near a thick wooden table with a fireplace burning behind me. I had a goblet in my hand and was jovially toasting the folks around me. I wore a long leather skirt, a fluffy white blouse, and a leather vest. My hair was brown and cut plainly in a medium-short length. There was no doubt that it was me. It did come as a surprise that I had apparently transcended time and had been a woman in a previous life."

There are hundreds of stories that go with regressions. Sorry I could not fit them all into this book.

Conclusion

**Hypnotherapy is an incredible tool,
just as the human mind and body are remarkable unto themselves.
Each of us is endowed with unlimited God given
potential, abilities, and possibilities.
Let's commit to use them to their fullest!**

Acknowledgements

Some of the ideas, inductions and suggestions in this book were adapted directly from the works of the following experts:

Raymond Moody

John G. Kappas

Josie Hadley

Carol Staudacher

Al Krasner

Deepak Chopra

Many, many thanks to them for their teachings and work in Quantum Physics, Healing, Philosophy, and Hypnotherapy!

Some Artwork by Jim Warren

Bibliography

Professional Hypnotism Manual
John G. Kappas

Hypnosis for Change
Josie Hadley and Carol Staudacher

The Book of Stress Survival
Alix Kirsta

The Journey Within
Henry Leo Bolduc

Magic Minute of Self Hypnosis
Mike Harvey

Past Life Regression
Barrie Konicov

Many Lives, Many Masters
Brian Weiss

Past Life Regression Guidebook
Bettye B. Binder

Life After Life
Raymond Moody

Ageless Mind, Timeless Body
Deepak Chopra

Perfect Health
Deepak Chopra

Quantum Physics
Deepak Chopra

The Wizard Within
Al Krasner

Clinical Hypnosis
Harold B. Crasilneck, James A. Hall

About The Author

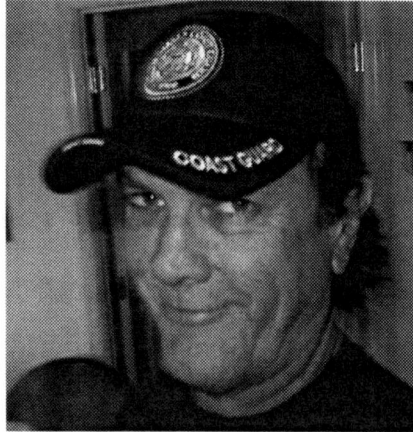

A native North Carolinian, Dr. Randall Maynard has lived in four countries, traveled the world extensively, and is multi-lingual.

He has studied and practiced Hypnotherapy for over 26 years. His clients have included professional Ice Hockey players and teams, golfers, the National Women's Tae Kwon Do Champion, The U.S. Olympic figure skating team, Colleges, Universities, Businesses, Civic organizations and individuals in all walks of life.

He holds a Ph.D. in Philosophy, a Masters in Clinical Hypnotherapy, and a Bachelors Degree in Psychology.

He is a U. S. Coast Guard Captain, a PADI certified open water diver, avid shark and Marlin fisherman, white water kayaker, racquetball player, accomplished musician, and former Hockey coach.

Dr. Maynard has been a public speaker for over 20 years and presents all of his programs in an interesting, unique, unexpected, and upbeat manner.

Email today to book him at your next event!

Nordique_1@msn.com

Web pages: www.attitude1.net

Ask about his retreats in SW Virginia, Norfolk, Va., and Stokesdale, N.C.

Publications By Dr. Maynard

Mind Games for Consenting Adults: 2nd Edition (Book)

Street Spanish (Text Book)

Superbolic Metabolism: Healing Via Cell Memory (CD)

John's Rules (Book))

Stress Management (CD)

Shamanic Voyaging (CD)

Behind The Mask (Hockey Goalie Article)

Smoking Cessation (CD)

The Juxtaposition Conspiracy (Article)

Can CNN Cause Cancer? (Article)

Buy Into It (article)

You Bet Your Life (Article)

Squirrel Busters (Article)

Weight Management (CD)

More…

Never Been Convicted (Autobiography)

Coming Soon: *The Hypnotist (Novel)*

What have you got to lose?

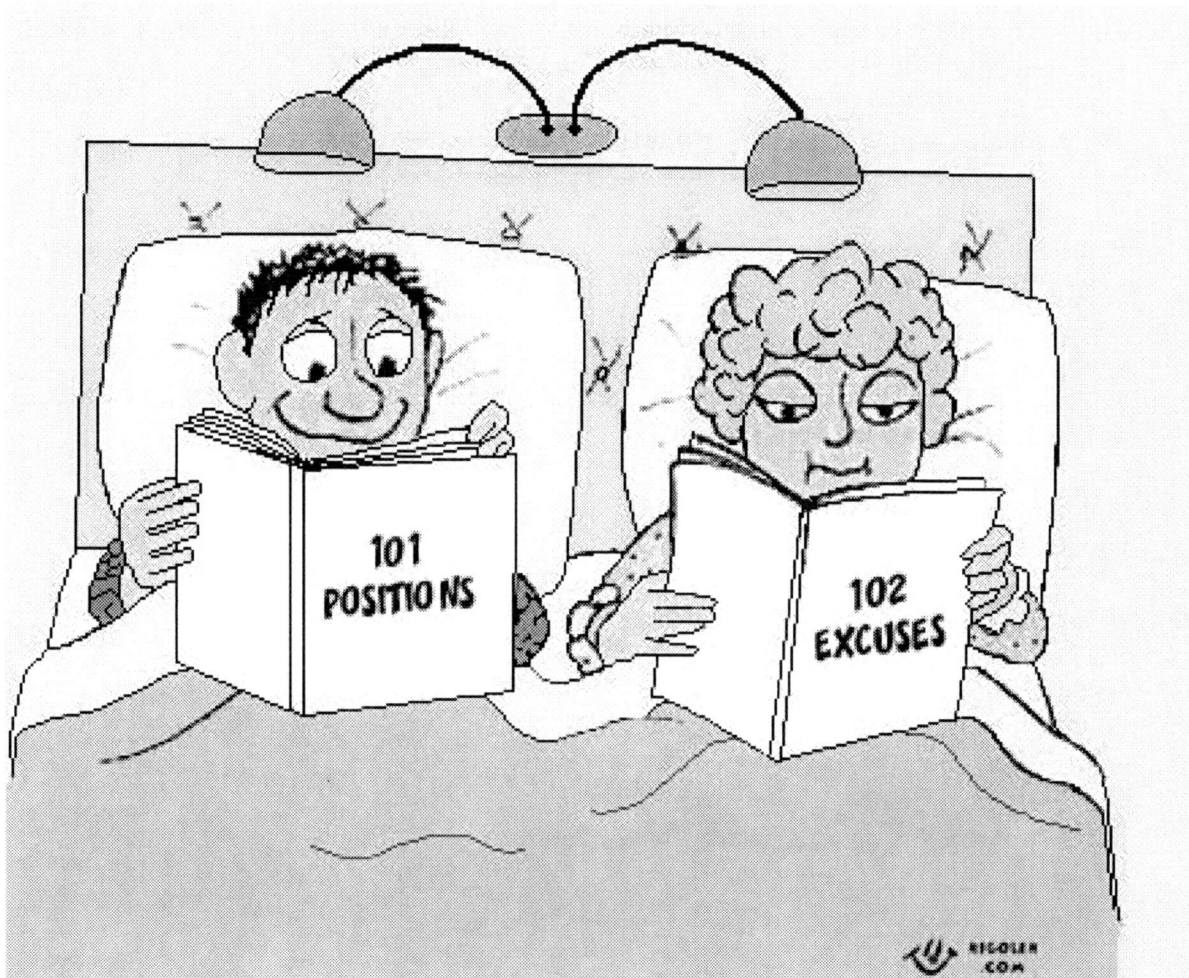

Addendum

There are literally thousands of possibilities for using Hypnosis/Hypnotherapy beyond those noted in this book.

If you can imagine it, it is possible.

There are many potential concepts ranging from Pain Management to Healing, Childbirth to Dental Fears, Bed wetting to Addiction Survival.

There are also many excellent Hypnotherapists available to assist you. Be sure to get proper referrals and credentials if and when you select one.

If you have not seen a Hypnotist stage show, you should. It will attack your funny bone from all angles.

God gave you unbelievable abilities when you were created. Hypnotherapy, properly applied, can help you discover many of them. Remember, your mind is very powerful and your only limits are you imagination.

A point to ponder…there are over 20,000 cases of cancer in remission using ONLY hypnotherapy as the treatment.

What else can you do with it?

Just imagine…..

My best wishes to you for a healthy, happy future!

Randy

Lightning Source UK Ltd.
Milton Keynes UK
11 February 2010

149915UK00001B/55/A

9 780615 140797